THE
JUST DIAGNOSED
GUIDE

HOW TO SUPPORT SOMEONE WHO'S SICK

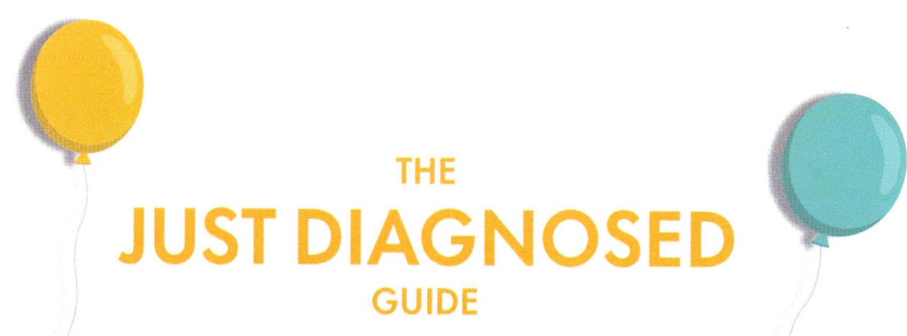

HOW TO SUPPORT SOMEONE WHO'S SICK

What You Need to Know Now (without Googling it)

JEN SINGER

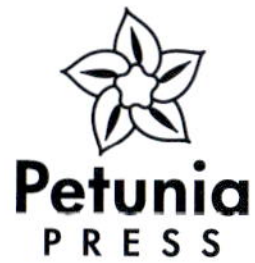

Red Bank, New Jersey

 Printed in the United States of America by Petunia Press, a division of MommaSaid, LLC, Red Bank, New Jersey.

Paperback ISBN: 979-8-9864391-7-4
Kindle ISBN: 979-8-9864391-3-6

DISCLAIMER:
FOR EDUCATIONAL AND INFORMATIONAL PURPOSES ONLY.

The author of this book is not a doctor, nurse, or any other type of medical professional. All content and information in this book are for informational and educational purposes only and do not constitute medical advice. The information provided is not a substitute for your doctor's care and does not attempt to diagnose, treat, prevent, or cure any physical, mental, or emotional condition. Please consult with your health care provider before taking any action or if you have any questions or concerns about your medical care, strategies, and options.

Contents

Just Diagnosed: How to Support Someone Who's Sick

Someone in your circle has been diagnosed with the kind of medical condition that makes people say, "Oh, damn."

Cancer. Heart failure. ALS. AIDS. Coronary artery disease. Pulmonary embolism. Parkinson's disease. Long Covid. Any of the "biggies."

What should you say?

What are you going to do to help?

If you're like most people, you might bake them a lasagna or send a Get Well card. You might remind them to "stay strong and be positive" and assure them that you'll keep them in your prayers. Maybe you'll even visit them in the hospital or start a GoFundMe campaign to cover their medical bills.

As someone who's been sick quite a bit, I can tell you that these might be perfectly fine attempts to support some-one who's just been diagnosed. But you're not looking for "perfectly fine." You want to do right by this person who's been dealt crappy cards and you don't want to say something wrong.

I've had loads of people say, "Oh, damn" about my diagnoses. At 40, I had an aggressive cancer. At 53, I had "Covid Classic" in the early days of the pandemic and soon, the electrical system of my heart began to shut down, leaving me with a pacemaker and heart failure.

Oh. Damn.

I know it's hard to figure out how to support someone who's sick because I've seen so many people try to do it for me. Some hit the mark. They organized playdates and rides to swim team practice for my kids, sent me chocolate and a cozy blanket for my Covid quarantine, and sat with me and my grief without trying to fix it or tsk-tsk it away.

Others, not so much. One person told me I'd attracted cancer with my thoughts. One told me her father had had the same diagnosis, but the cancer didn't kill him. "The chemo did." One insisted that my heart failure would "reverse itself" into a spontaneous and miraculous healing, even though that's not exactly the prognosis my cardiologist gave me.

It's not enough to mean well. It's time we all do it well, too.

Whenever it's my turn to support someone else who's sick, I try to remember that there are two major rules of being a patient:

1. *What they need logistically changes.*
2. *What they need emotionally doesn't.*

As a society, we tend to be very good at logistics. We deliver dinners, pick up prescriptions, and take the patient to chemo or doctor's appointments. We send flowers, post updates on private Facebook pages, and make Target runs.

But emotional support is much harder to supply because most of us have been taught how to do it all wrong. Many people think their job is to cheer up the patient, lofting platitudes that we've all been taught to say:

"God only gives us what we can handle."

"Everything happens for a reason."

"That which doesn't kill you...."

What? Mutates and comes back to try again?

In all my years of being sick, I've learned how to support someone who's sick. I'm going to make it easier for you to do it, because that's all we desperately want to do when a family member, friend, neighbor, or acquaintance gets an "oh, damn" diagnosis. We just need to learn a few things first.

So go ahead and bake that lasagna, send flowers, or pick up your visitor's badge at the hospital's front desk. But there's so much more to supporting someone's who's sick, and you're about to find out how, you healthcare hero, you.

Thank you for being there when we need you the most.

When Someone Gets a Big Diagnosis

At 7:30 on a Tuesday morning, my brother suddenly appeared in the doorway of my hospital room on the oncology floor at New York-Presbyterian on Manhattan's Upper East Side.

"Scott? Why are you here?"

"I'm on my way to work," he said.

"But you live in New Jersey and you work in New Jersey." He wasn't on his way to anything. He'd braved rush hour traffic across the George Washington Bridge because he'd decided I needed a visitor during my first five-day infusion of chemotherapy for stage III non-Hodgkin's lymphoma. My young sons were home with their father, getting ready for their final days in the second and third grades. I longed to be home with them, packing lunches, and scouring their rooms for overdue library books.

Scott was right. I needed a visitor and that visitor needed to be him. That he was holding my new iPod full of some two hundred songs he'd loaded for me was the bonus prize. That one of the songs was "Just the Two of Us" by Dr. Evil with Mini Me from "Austin Powers" was pure genius.

Some people just instinctively know how to support someone who's sick. Scott knew how to support me. When I was diagnosed, we had been in the middle of a years-long "Extreme Quarterly Lunch" tradition, when we alternated lunches at fine New York City restaurants and sticky-floored hot dog joints along New Jersey highways. So, one night during chemo, he brought me filet mignon from a chichi Manhattan restaurant and toasted me with ginger ale in four-ounce plastic hospital water cups.

But he wasn't the only one to support me in ways, big and small, that made it easier to endure my craptastic diagnosis:

- An anonymous neighbor found my son's flip-flops, marked SINGER in black Sharpie, on the beach at our community lake and stuck them in my mailbox instead of leaving them in the Lost and Found.
- A neighbor who owns a restaurant sent trays of food to the house, and my foodie son dropped everything to follow the delivery from the van to the dining room table.
- Friends and acquaintances sent toys and other goodies to my kids, and others delivered much-needed wine to my then-husband.
- Friends set up picnics in my hospital room.
- People sent heartfelt cards to let me know they were thinking of me.
- A dear friend sent one of my sons a New York Mets blanket and the other, a New York Yankees blanket. I'd

fall asleep on the couch under the Mets and wake up under the Yankees and vice-versa.

If actions speak louder than words, I was getting some pretty loud love. I was so very lucky. The luck continued after my heart failure diagnosis in 2020, back when we were all trapped in our houses learning how to make sourdough starter and not kill each other.

It seemed like every week another package appeared on my porch. Friends near and far—it didn't matter where they were because we couldn't get together—sent me all sorts of treats to let me know they were thinking of me and my new pacemaker and the fact that I would never play tennis again. Here's just some of what they sent:

- Several T-shirts featuring my Facebook post sign-off, "Stay gold, Pony Boy"
- Easter chocolates shaped like bunnies
- Various masks, some with fancy writing to disguise curse words
- An "Oodie," which is an oversized wearable blanket that I wore both inside and outside the house, because it made people cross the street to avoid me, taking their cooties with them
- Not one, but two bracelets that read, "You fucking got this"
- A Timex watch because I "take a licking and keep on ticking"
- A Wonder Woman logo hood ornament
- An ebook about the history of the heart
- A red cape

- Gift baskets full of food
- Cat toys for my Benny

There was the stuff, sure, but there was also plenty of moral support. It felt like everyone was collectively holding space for my grief. They didn't try to fix the problem or talk me out of my sadness for what I'd lost or what I feared might happen.

Best of all, they didn't "other" me. That's when people feel sorry for the patient, treating them with pity more than empathy. Brené Brown calls pity a "near enemy" of compassion. It's an "oh this bad thing happened to you but will never happen to me" kind of attitude.

I suppose I didn't get as much pity in 2020 as I did with cancer because everyone was scared shitless they, too, would get Covid and end up in a bad way. Well, most everyone. There was some "othering" because I'd had a pre-existing condition that led to heart failure. Or as I like to say, cancer treatments filled the barn with dynamite and Covid lit the match.

But nobody blamed my thoughts or pushed me to be positive, and that was welcomed with giant Oodie arms.

Patients don't need pity. We need compassion and empathy and maybe a good friend to check our torso for EKG electrodes.

What Not to Say When Someone's Sick

Generally speaking, we are terrible at cheering people up when they're sick. There's a reason for that:

IT ISN'T OUR JOB TO CHEER THEM UP.

I don't know how it started, but someone, somewhere decided that when a family member, friend, or acquaintance tells you they're sick with one of those "oh damn" diagnoses, we are supposed to get them to look on the bright side. It's like we're photographers holding up shiny objects to coax children to smile for the picture. Quick! Get the bubbles! Someone stopped smiling!

Here's what we might say:

"Stay strong and be positive."

"Everything happens for a reason."

"There are people who have it worse than you do."

"It's always darkest before the dawn."

"God only gives you what you can handle."

"That which doesn't kill you makes you stronger."

These might seem like reasonable things to say, but I'm telling you as a person who has had not one, but two life-threatening diseases, they not only don't help, they can actually hurt. Here's why:

"Stay strong and be positive." If you've ever had cancer, it's likely you've heard this one. It isn't a friendly bon mot so much as it's homework because it implies that your attitude will cure your cancer, and that is patently false.

The American Cancer Society reports that studies have proven that maintaining a positive attitude doesn't "change the course of a person's cancer" or extend lives. Rather, it can make patients feel guilty about their very valid feelings of fear, sadness, and anxiety. I mean, if you can't feel bad when you have freakin' cancer, when can you?

I've also seen it exchanged among heart condition patients and that's more complicated, because there are studies tying optimism to a reduction in the risk for heart disease. It's true that negative emotions can release stress hormones that can raise blood pressure.

You know what's really stressful, though? When you're scared because you have a pacemaker surgery coming up or worried that you won't be able to keep up with your family on vacation and then someone chastises you with,

"You have to be positive!" Now you're not only scared or worried, you're also feeling guilty because you can't turn that frown upside-down, ya big Eeyore, you.

The bottom line: Don't tell people how they should feel, even if you've been in their shoes. Everybody does disease differently, and it isn't for us to dictate how.

"Everything happens for a reason." This is the sort of thing that gets needlepointed onto pillows. I blame Michael J. Fox.

In his memoir, "Lucky Man," Fox wrote, "Life is great. Sometimes, though, you just have to put up with a little more crap." For a while there, he was the poster boy for optimism in the face of an "oh damn" diagnosis, and he's surely been an inspiration for my mom since she got Parkinson's.

But that bright-sided heroism became the hot thing for far too long. It might be why a friend posted on my Facebook wall that I was "supposed to get cancer" so that I can help people by writing about my experience. No thanks. I'd rather have a reason for writing about surfing or gardening or Netflix.

But we create reason; it doesn't happen to us. Fox turned his lemons into an incredible foundation to raise money for Parkinson's disease research, largely because he had the means, the platform, and the drive. In a later memoir, though, he said he was "out of the lemonade business" after a tumor on his spine left him stranded on his kitchen floor while home alone. That's more than "a little more crap," thank you very much. Like most of us, he felt different things at different stages of disease, and managed to find purpose along the way.

Whether "everything happens for a reason" is meant as a religious or spiritual surrender or a directive to make lemonade, it usually doesn't make the patient feel better.

But ice cream generally does. I like rainbow sprinkles on mine.

"There are people who have it worse than you do." In other words, suck it up, Buttercup. It could be worse and therefore, you have no reason to complain.

I'm not advocating for whining, but I do think it's okay to feel bad about feeling bad, even if there are other people who feel worse than you. I was aware that there were sicker cancer patients than me because I had several hospital roommates who were dying. But I was 40 years-old and I had a tumor the size of a softball in my left lung. While all the other moms were at my kid's Little League game, I was in my hospital bed swishing "magic mouthwash" over the sores the chemo left in my throat. That sucks, and it's okay to say so, even in real time.

"It's always darkest before the dawn." In other words, it's always the worst right before it gets better. It's like saying "Hang in there" and "You can do it!" It may seem like benign cheerleading, except there's a problem with it: Sometimes, things don't get better. If, for instance, you have a chronic condition, it may get bad and then worse and then okay and then truly horrible before leveling out again.

I had a curable cancer, so I could psyche myself up for chemo knowing I'd feel worse before I felt better—again and again—for six rounds of chemo and five weeks of radiation treatments. But heart failure isn't like that. It's a chronic condition that feels like I'm playing a cruel game of Chutes & Ladders. I've fluctuated between stage 2 and 3 and back again. I've felt great for weeks and then ended up in the ER, escorted via wheelchair from cardiac rehab in a T-shirt that suddenly seemed really stupid to wear in public: "Call in Seasick."

Sometimes it's darkest before the dawn. Sometimes it's just plain dark.

"God only gives you what you can handle." This came from the same chuckle patch as "Everything happens for a reason." It implies that you cannot break down into a puddle of tears upon getting a harrowing diagnosis because a higher being has chosen you as the next Job. If you endure this particular obstacle course, you'll win eternal life in the good seats in Heaven or at least the spotlight when the deejay plays "I Will Survive" at your niece's wedding.

But you have to *handle* it. And by handle it, what's really meant is that you must keep a stiff upper lip and be positive and stay strong and find meaning in your trauma, perhaps by sharing your sob story on "The Voice" and then getting a record deal. Or something like that.

God absolutely gives us more than we can handle. That's why there's a Suicide Hotline. Telling someone this platitude is akin to saying, "You'll be fine and I don't want to hear about your icky problem anymore." Or it's like saying, "Only a higher power can help you now. See ya."

Don't emotionally abandon the patient.

"That which doesn't kill you makes you stronger." This springs from the patient-as-hero myth that's based on the idea that we've been through some pretty awful things, so clearly, we must have earned the wisdom of Yoda and the strength of the Hulk.

Maybe. But maybe we have neuropathy, cataracts, and a touch of PTSD from what we've been through, too. Maybe just getting enough energy and interest to attend the weekly status meeting at work is all we can summon in lieu of a dissertation on the meaning of life.

Look, I'm grateful to be alive and I've learned to let go of a lot of nonsense I no longer tolerate since Death rang my doorbell—twice. But sometimes, the wisest thing I can do is remember to defrost the chicken in time to cook it for dinner.

Am I stronger? Depends on what you mean. I used to be able to bench press 75 pounds and now I have to think twice about carrying in an Amazon box from the porch, lest I wind up wheeling toward the ER again. I'd rather have my gym membership and my muscle tone back than whatever this brand of strength is.

Wait. Then What *Do* We Say to People Who Are Sick?

We were driving around Wildwood, New Jersey, trying to find a parking spot near an ice cream parlor (hello, sprinkles!) when my cell phone rang. It was a friend I hadn't yet talked to since my cancer diagnosis two chemo rounds earlier. I let it go to voicemail, and then I made a big mistake: I listened to it.

"Hi, Jen. I am so devastated by your cancer diagnosis. I am so very sorry. You must be scared. And the kids? Oh my God. When do you go to chemo next? Anyhow, give me a call back when you get a chance."

I was on vacation, thinking only about my mocha chip ice cream with rainbow sprinkles and my sons' wonderful, messy, melty cones we were about to get, and now, suddenly, I was pulled right back into the shitshow my life had become that summer. Worse, I was now holding space for the well-meaning friend's devastation at *my* diagnosis.

We can do better. I'm on a mission to help us all do that.

Remember when I said that what sick people need emotionally doesn't change? Do you wonder what they need from you? It's what we all need when we're in crisis:

Empathy and validation.

How do you deliver that? By listening.

Now, don't flip the page because you assume you know how to listen. I've been studying and practicing listening skills for over a decade and I still have things to learn. And I don't just mean, put down your phone and look them in the eyes, though that's a good start. I mean *active listening*, because it meets the patient where they are and makes them feel heard.

I'm going to give you six words you can say to anyone at any point in their healthcare wild ride (it's not a journey) that's infused with empathy:

"How is it for you today?"

Then zip your lips and listen. Whatever comes out of their mouth is not for you to:

1. *fix*
2. *judge*
3. *distract them from*
4. *tell them you know what they mean because your uncle had the same thing and he died from it (and therefore, he had it worse, so be grateful)*

5. *insert your vaguely related story or more harrowing experience, thereby hijacking the theme of how it is for them today*
6. *make them take care of your emotions*

"How is it today" makes room for whatever they might need from you, if anything because—and this is the important part—you are going to validate it.

If, for instance, they say, "I'm really worried about my next round of chemo," you would encourage them to tell you more about why just by letting them talk. And then you might say one of two phrases:

> "No wonder...."
>
> "Of course...."
>
> "No wonder you're worried. It sounds like the first round was really hard."
>
> "Of course you're worried. The side effects sound awful."

Then be quiet and let them say whatever comes to them next.

How might this have worked if I'd picked up the phone during our ice cream run?

> "How is it for you today?"

"We're on vacation down the shore and getting ice cream. I'm glad not to deal with doctors or chemo right now."

> "Of course you're glad! What a great treat to be on vacation with your family in the middle of all this!"

"We practically poured me into my mini-van from my hospital room, but I made it! And Chris has chocolate sprinkles running down his arm right now."

That's meeting the patient where they are because that's how it was for me that day.

You might wonder what my friend could have left on my voicemail when I didn't pick up. How about:

> "I heard about your cancer diagnosis and I'm calling to see how it is for you today. Call back whenever you feel like it—or not. Just know I'm thinking of you."

See the difference?

Start simply with active listening, which combines empathy with validation, and you'll begin to truly support someone who's sick.

Why "If There's Anything I Can Do" Falls Short

You're finishing your conversation with someone who's sick, and you say what so many people say, "Let me know if there's anything I can do."

But this, too, is homework for the patient, because now, they've got to come up with some way you can help when they've got plenty on their plate already. And they've got to match it up to where you are in their Circles of Support:

Circles of Support

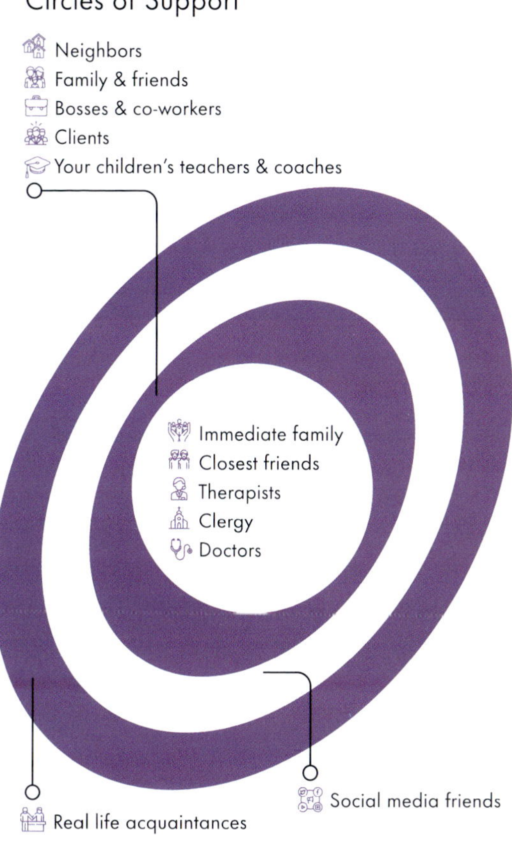

These circles matter because they give the patient a guideline to follow on what to share and with whom. If you're just someone they run into at school plays, for instance, you're going to be in an outer circle. But if you're on their emergency contact list, more will be expected—and welcomed—from you. If you're a social media friend, that's a different expectation altogether, unless, of course, you've had the same disease and can offer insights and knowing empathy that others can't.

So why can't you just say, "If there's anything I can do," no matter what circle you're in?

Imagine you've just come home from the hospital with a new "oh damn" diagnosis. Your significant other is out picking up your new prescriptions. Your teenager is bringing in the DoorDash delivery for dinner. Your next-door neighbor is putting a few groceries in your fridge. Your 10 year-old and your cat are snuggled up next to you as though they'll never let you leave again.

Someone calls. It's a friend whose sister had the same diagnosis as you. You talk about treatments and doctors as carefully as you can with your little one sitting next to you. The call comes to an end, but before she hangs up, she says, "If there's anything I can do..."

Now you've got to come up with something for her to do so that she feels helpful during your time of need. But what if she offered up some "anythings" instead?

> "If you'd like to talk to someone who's been through what you're about to go through, I can introduce you to my sister."
>
> "When my sister was sick, I did all the research on treatments and clinical trials. I'd be glad to cull it down to what you need to know and send it over, if you'd like."

> "I'm going to send you a blanket like the one my sister brought to chemo and some cool headscarves. Is that okay with you?"
>
> "I'm free to take you to your treatments next week if you'd like company."
>
> "I made banana bread. Would you like me to drop it off for breakfast? I can leave it in the mailbox so I don't bug anyone."

The more thinking you can do, the less work it is for the patient. If you're not sure what to do, ask other people in your Circle of Support for suggestions. Another good place to check is the patient support website or private Facebook page, if one has been set up. If there isn't one, maybe you could be the one to create it (but ask first).

Isn't There Anything I Can Do?

Yes, there's absolutely something you can do. It all depends on what the patient needs, where you are in the Circles of Support, where you live relative to the patient, and what resources, such as money, time, or ground transportation, you have.

To support someone who's sick, you can do stuff, buy stuff, or say stuff.

Do Stuff

The obvious "do" is helping with day-to-day logistics. This is often the most satisfying way to help because it's a tangible assist, chipping in when life goes sideways for someone you care about. Here's some stuff you can do:

Organize the doing – When I had cancer, one close friend maintained a schedule for dinner donations from neighbors so that we wouldn't wind up with three lasagnas in a row. This was especially helpful because we'd gutted our kitchen in a remodel right when I was diagnosed. Lucky for us, neighbors would drop off their designated meal according to the schedule, so we only needed the microwave and the fridge which had been temporarily relocated to the dining room.

Cook – When the healthy get sick, the chefs get cooking. In so many cultures, food is love, so what better way to show you care than cooking? But before you drop off your favorite casserole, keep a few things in mind:

- **Don't use your own dishes.** I wound up with a box full of my neighbors' dishes and pots and I had no idea who they belonged to. Make it easier on everyone and use disposable, yet reusable, containers. If you must use your own dishes, affix a label with your name and number on them before you drop off dinner and then arrange to pick them back up.
- **What the patient can eat may change.** Naturally, you should cook with the patient's allergies and food preferences in mind. But understand that what they can eat may change with treatments. Chemo can leave painful ulcers in the mouth and radiation can make it hard to swallow. Cardiac patients may have limits on their sodium and fat intake, and patients on blood thinners may have to cut out vitamin K, which is prevalent in spinach, kale, and green tea. Ask about any restrictions.
- **Time it right.** Everybody wants to cook for the patient during the first weeks after a diagnosis. As a result, they can wind up with food they can't eat and a stuffed freezer. Consider cooking after the initial rush ends.
- **Drop-off information.** Suggest or offer up a cooler they can leave outside their house in case they are not home to receive meals. It will also keep the racoons

away. But make sure they know there is food there, so it doesn't rot.

Be Uber – Cart the patient to appointments and procedures, which may be frequent. For instance, radiation treatments tend to be scheduled at the same time every weekday, for multiple weeks. Chemotherapy can take place as often as weekly, and dialysis can occur several times a week or even several times a day. Cardiac rehab and physical therapy are often several times a week. You can offer to drop the patient off or, depending on the visitor rules, keep them company at their appointment. Let the patient decide.

Consider setting up an easy way for them to ask for rides so they don't feel like they're bothering anyone, especially if they live alone or with minor children. For example, you could set up a calendar on a patient care site or a private Facebook page just for rides.

My hospital offered a free ride service after my pacemaker surgery, but I wasn't allowed to go alone, or else the driver would have liability for my woozy, post-op self. My son would have to ride with me. We took the ferry instead—fewer bumps and no erratic New York/New Jersey drivers along the way.

If the patient has kids, they still need to get to their usual activities. One of my neighbors set up a carpool schedule so that my sons would get to swim team practice and meets, and to plenty of playdates during the summer I was in chemo.

Keep the home running – Do laundry, run errands, clean the house, do the dishes, mow the lawn, shovel the walk, feed the pets, or walk the dog. If you're handy, fix things. Pay the bills, sign the kids up for activities by the deadlines, and stock the pantry.

It's helpful to keep their homes in season because it maintains some semblance of normalcy. You can offer to do things like putting up or taking down holiday decorations, bringing out the deck furniture, or stacking up wood by the fireplace.

Set up a medical fundraising site – In this era of medical debt, helping the patient offset the costs of treatment (or supplementing income if they can't work during treatment) is the ultimate "do." But only if the patient wants you to set it up. Ideally, this should be handled by someone in the patient's inner circle.

Be sure to set it up so the funds transfer goes directly to the patient's bank account. It will require some work on their part, or on yours if they trust you with their banking information. Be very clear about what you're raising the money for because people often prefer to donate to a specific bill or goal and be sure to update and thank donors regularly.

Buy Stuff

You can offer everything from the practical to the silly. Buying stuff for the patient is about what they need logistically as well as emotionally.

I've been gifted headscarves and hats, blankets and gift baskets, a series of silly wigs and a Barbie "doodle board," which I used to report my pain levels to my nurse, Robert, who looked like Benjamin Bratt and brought me my prescription pain meds. I was a fan of Robert.

If you're thinking of sending something to the patient, ask yourself these questions:

Does it make them work for it? It does if it requires assembly, they have to be home to sign for it, they have to figure out something technical (and that's not their jam), or it's loud and/or leaves a mess.

Is everyone else sending the same thing right now? Everyone wants to be the one who delivers dinner the night the patient gets home from the hospital. It's the glory meal that gets a shout-out on social media: *Stacey is home from surgery and enjoying the chicken piccata that the Pattersons dropped off. Thank you!* But not everyone can be the Pattersons, and the patient is going to need food after her 19th radiation treatment, too.

Will it make them smile? There's nothing quite like the feeling you get when you've spent the week facing needles and big, scary medical machinery and you get something thoughtful from someone who cares. I imagine it's like a message from earth when you thought your spaceship had spun out of orbit forever. Thank you, thank you, thank you for making us smile.

About Gift Cards

Gift cards are always a good way to go. Consider gift cards for food delivery from local restaurants or services like Seamless or Instacart. One friend even set up an old school account at a local deli which I used for lunch (and sometimes also dinner) on long summer days. Here are some other gift card ideas:

- gasoline, ride share, or train/bus/ferry
- bookstores
- coffee shops
- ice cream shops
- toys for their kids and/or pets
- big box stores or Amazon where they can get all sorts of items
- music
- clothing
- streaming video sites
- spa or massage (Note that cancer patients may not be allowed to get manicures or pedicures during treatments because they can lead to infections in immunocompromised patients.)
- Visa/Mastercard-type gift cards

Consider buying things to entertain the patient's kids, such as board or video games, books, or gift cards for movie downloads. (Tip: The 1968 film, "Chitty Chitty Bang Bang" is 2 hours and 25 nap-worthy minutes long.) Be sure not to send anything loud, messy, or made up of thousands of pieces, or something that requires assembly or constant supervision. For the love of all that's holy, please don't send anything that might land someone in the ER. (I'm looking at you, pogo sticks.)

Also, think through your selection from the patient's point of view. I was between chemo five and six when I summoned up the energy to play a board game with the kids. What did they choose? The game of Life. So now I'm driving a plastic car full of pink and blue "children" toward "retirement" when in real life, I wasn't even sure if I'd make it past Christmas. I tried to sell them on Candy Land and even Sorry! but alas.

Say Stuff

One of the most helpful things you can do for a patient is to be their advocate. Or, as my brother calls it, their Medical Enforcer. This is the person who stands up to doctors, nurses, hospital administrators, and health insurance companies to ensure the best care and most affordable coverage that the patient can get.

It takes a particular set of skills to perform this role well, some of which you'll learn on the job. But it helps if you have some sort of medical background, either as a patient or a healthcare worker. Good research skills are a must because you might need to sift through medical papers, read insurance plans, hunt down top doctors and hospitals, and decipher Explanation of Benefits and bills.

In short, you become the patient's voice when they need it most. What does it look like? Here are a few examples of my own Medical Enforcing:

> After a knee replacement, my mother had a side effect from anesthesia that sometimes affects the elderly:

> hallucinations. Her doctor wanted to release her from the hospital, but I persuaded him not to send her home to my father, who was in his 80s, while she still asking when it would stop raining worms outside.
>
> I knew enough not to pay the full estimated amount for my pacemaker surgery the morning of, despite the pressure to do so. Instead, I negotiated a smaller down payment, which is some darn good Medical Enforcing for myself.
>
> When the veterinarian (yes, pets count here) asked me to bring my cat, Benny in for testing to determine if we should increase his insulin dosage for diabetes, I said no. Benny was dying of an aggressive cancer, and he hated going to the vet's office. Instead, I asked her what I should look for if he were to have a reaction to an increased dose. Then I gave him that dose and watched for symptoms. He tolerated it well, and we avoided future vet visits for the remainder of his life.

If you're going to speak directly to medical providers, insurance companies, and Medicare or Medicaid, the patient will need to sign HIPAA (Health Insurance Portability and Accountability Act) papers, which provide consent to share patient health information. Ask the doctor's office and hospital for the papers. Medicare has forms online.

If you accompany the patient to medical appointments, the patient may be able to verbally agree to name you as an advocate. Ask the doctor to add it to their patient record.

When Their Diagnosis Affects You

If you're in the patient's inner circle, it's likely that their diagnosis is having a significant impact on your life. Whether the patient is a spouse or partner, a parent or child, a sibling or other family member, a close friend, a business partner, or even a fellow youth sports coach or volunteer, your day-to-day life is now affected—and so are your heart and soul.

Many people in a patient's inner circle instinctively stuff their feelings, figuring that their worry, fear, and sadness pale in comparison to the patient's. But I'm telling you as a patient who has had many Circles of Support, your emotions matter.

Let me say it out loud right *to* you:

"No wonder you feel the way you do."

"Of course you feel that way."

This. Is. Hard.

In the beginning, you might get swooped up in a swirl of adrenaline as you jump in to handle the logistics in your corner of this battle. This is the "fight" part of "fight, flight, or freeze," and it can be heady. You might feel like you're part of a formidable team that's going to help save the patient. And you just might be.

So go ahead and schedule appointments, deliver food, fill your basket at CVS or Walmart, and go, fight, win! But in the wee hours of the night, in the moments of solitude in the shower or in your car, deep down in your head when things quiet down, listen to that little voice inside you. Is it scared? Is it angry at God? At the illness? At the doctors? Do you feel guilty because you're healthy and yet, you can't do it all yourself? Do you have a mish-mosh of feelings you can't sort out?

Let me ask you a question: How is it for you today? Really, I mean it. How is it? Do you feel like you can't tell the patient how you really are? When people stop you in parking lots and lobbies to ask, "How are you holding up?" do you tell the truth? Or are you deliberately pushing aside your needs because you, quite understandably, must tend to the patient, logistically and emotionally?

That takes its toll, and then you can wind up being useless to the patient or yourself. Here in the patient's inner circle, you must carve out what you need to restore and refresh. Start by acknowledging and validating your own feelings. "Of course....no wonder....". Then take deliberate and active steps to support yourself and to accept support from others. Here are a few tips:

Breathe. No, really. When we're stressed we tend to hold our breath, which can shift us into "fight-or-flight" mode by releasing cortisol, a hormone that can increase blood sugar levels and make the heart work harder. Make sure you're "belly breathing," filling your lungs with air as though you're trying to fill your stomach like a balloon. Five breaths in and five breaths out can help you reset.

Get help for the helpers. You know all those people who said, "If there's anything I can do..."? Give them something to do. Let them take over something that you have limited time and energy for. If you live with the patient, let someone else handle some of the day-to-day logistics of running the household. You don't have to be the one who always takes the patient for tests or treatments and, if you play your cards right, you might not have to cook for a long time.

If you're currently running a company without your business partner because of illness, consider leaning on other leaders or even bringing in a temporary manager to fill in. If you're coaching a team or running a volunteer position without your partner, ask someone to help, even if you wind up with rotating assistant coaches, Scout leaders, or class parents. Someone else can remember to bring the soccer balls for a while. You've got enough on your mind. Besides, people love to help. Give them something to do.

Keep something that's yours. You need something that helps you escape from all things medical. If the gym is where you get rid of your stress, keep on going. Keep running, playing cards, going to book club—whatever serves as a taste of normal in an otherwise irregular time. One caveat is booze or drugs. More might feel better in the moment, but we all know it's not a great escape in the long run.

Get support. Caregivers can suffer from burnout, especially if they've taken on most of the daily responsibilities. Consider joining a support group for caregivers or seeing a therapist.

Perhaps join *patient* support groups on social media, through hospital websites, or through organizations focusing on the specific condition, because you'll learn a lot from patients and you'll find other caregivers like you.

Think of yourself like a racecar. You can't keep zooming around the track without pulling into the pitstop for gas and new tires now and then. Supporters need support, too.

If you're the patient, consider giving your closest caregivers some care back. Here's how I did it:

When my son, Nick, dropped me off at the ER early in the pandemic, I worried about him. It was April 2020, and, thanks to Covid, he was finishing his senior year of art school online, in my dining room. He couldn't come into the hospital with me because of Covid restrictions, and frankly, I wouldn't want him to. He was an adult (just barely), but he wasn't ready to watch his mom get hooked up to a defibrillator just in case her heart went kaput.

As soon as I could, I started a text chain with the following inner circle people: the son in my house and the one up in Ithaca, my brother, and several of my closest friends. I had a separate text going with a friend who's also a nurse, so I wouldn't scare the civilians with the medical details. I asked everyone to watch over my kids because I knew this would dig up old feelings from when Mom was whisked away to a hospital in New York for half a summer when they were little.

And did they ever watch over them. They sent them both DoorDash gift cards and beer, and even took their dinner orders and sent food from local restaurants. They called to check in and to talk about what was going on. It was the support system they needed before they would take over supporting me. For two weeks, Nick dropped food outside my quarantine room, fed the cat, brought in the mail, and did the dishes. Chris finished up his junior year and came home, quarantining first in an Airbnb because we were pre-vaccine and I was high-risk.

Everyone who was taking care of me was taking care of each other. I realize that not everyone has that kind of kumbaya energy or network. But if the patient and their team, big or small, support each other even in little ways, the whole ordeal gets easier on everyone involved.

What Patients Want

I asked patients what others did for them that really stuck with them. Here's what they said:

"When I was going through chemo, one friend would make plans to just come sit on the couch and watch mindless television with me."

"When I was in the hospital and wasn't able to take a shower for nearly a week, my friend brought dry shampoo and helped me use it. It was one of the kindest things anyone has ever done for me."

"After my mastectomy and radiation, I couldn't even pick up my baby for a while. Some old friends started showing up every day so I could nap. They were aware that I was feeling like a failure as a mom, but there was no judgment."

"My neighbor played with my exercise-starved dog outside, even though she wasn't really a dog person."

"Simply being present with me in the ICU so I wasn't alone."

"When I was in the hospital on Thanksgiving, my friends cooked a whole Thanksgiving meal and brought it to me with pretty plates and some little gifts. So nice of them!"

"Someone made a 'When you are better jar.' People wrote down something they would do with me when I got out of the hospital and put it in the jar. It gave me something to look forward to."

"Said the Mi Shebeirach." (Jewish prayer for healing.)

"I'm single, so having someone to drive me to surgery, stay with me until it was safe for me to be alone, and walk my dog was helpful."

"When I was going through chemo and radiation, one of my friends simply listened to me. She didn't make suggestions. She didn't judge me. She simply let me talk. She simply let me be—and I can't tell you what a rare and precious gift that was."

"Asking what would be most helpful to me in the moment, and then continuing to ask once in a while."

"My husband sat with me and held my hand. He cried when I cried from the pain but never tried to hush me. He never tried to tell me it would get better. He never walked away from my suffering. He simply let me release and let me know I was loved."

Platitude Substitutions

I've given you some phrases to say to begin to actively listen to the patient:

"How is it for you today?"

"No wonder..." or "Of course..."

Now let's start replacing those worn-out platitudes with phrases that truly support someone who's sick.

Old: "You have to be positive and stay strong!"

New: "This is a tough thing to go through. I'll be with you along the way."

Old: "Everything happens for a reason."

New: "This sucks. I'm going to drop off some (insert item or food)."

Old: "Other people have it worse than you."

New: "I know this is hard on you. Can I make it a little easier by (fill in with clever thing to do, buy, or say)?"

Old: "It's always darkest before the dawn."

New: "The ups and downs can be too much. What's the worst of it for you right now?" Then listen and validate! (e.g. "No wonder you're worried about that procedure.")

Old: "God only gives you what you can handle."

New: "I can take you to your scan next week, and, if you're up for it, we'll stop at the diner after."

Old: "That which doesn't kill you makes you stronger."

New: "Some days are going to be really hard. I'm sending some emergency chocolate (or whatever they can eat)."

Old: "Let me know if there's anything I can do."

New: "I'm not entirely sure what you need from me, but I can cook dinner on Sunday night, send groceries via Instacart, read you a book, create a personalized playlist for your treatments, or scream into pillows with you. Patient's choice."

Holding Space

If you begin to actively listen, the patient will likely feel safe enough to open up and share how they really feel.

If the thought of that terrifies you, you might want to avoid letting the conversation get too deep. You can say, "Of course you feel that way" and then segue into an offer to send over some brownies or something.

But if you're willing and able to hold space for whatever's on the patient's mind—and I mean, *whatever*—then be prepared to listen and validate, over and over. Here's how that might look:

> You: "How is it for you today?"
> Patient: "I'm not good...." (begins to cry)
> You: "You're not good." (Repeating what they say shows you heard them without editorializing, fixing, or distracting them. Just don't sound like a disinterested parrot.)
> Patient: "No...it's...I know I should be grateful to be alive, but I'm scared..."
> You: "Of course you're scared. This is hard. What's the worst of it right now?" (You didn't guess why they were scared or talk them out of it. You stayed curious. Good on you.)

> Patient: "I'm scared I won't be around to see the kids graduate from high school."

Did alarm bells just go off in your head and heart? Quick! Get the bubbles! Someone stopped smiling.

Many people will respond to such a heavy realization this way:

"Don't say that! The doctors are doing all they can, and you're strong. You'll beat this!"

In just three sentences, they've shut down the patient's true feelings, chastised them, gave them homework, and ignored reality. No wonder being a patient can feel so lonely, even when you're surrounded by people who love you and mean well.

If, however, you're willing to continue to hold space for the patient, here's how the conversation might go:

> Patient: "I'm scared I won't be around to see the kids graduate from high school."
> You: "There's a part of you that's scared you won't be here. Is that right?" (Using the phrase "part of you" helps separate out the fear.)
> Patient: "I can't tell my husband that. He gets mad at me."
> You: "He can't hear that right now." (This is validation with slightly different wording. The "right now" part reminds the patient that this isn't forever.)

Patient: "No. But...I. What if the treatments don't work?"
You: "Is it okay to let that scared part of you know that we're here, and we're listening?"
Patient: "Yes." (Deep breath.) "I feel silly bringing this up. I mean, my last scan was better."
You: "Yet that part of you still worries."
Patient: "Yes! It's like a lifeguard, scanning the waves for trouble."
You: "How about we let it do its job while we go for a walk, if you're up for it? Or maybe we can watch 'Ferris Bueller's Day Off' for the bazillionth time?"
Patient: "Free Ferris!"
And scene.

You didn't try to talk them out of their feelings. You didn't try to fix it. You didn't insert your own story. You didn't give them homework. You didn't spout platitudes. You just did some active listening, and no doubt that scared part of them felt heard and validated.

Which means you may actually have cheered them up.

How about them apples?

Carry On, Healthcare Heroes

The fact that you've just read a book on how to support someone who's sick is proof that you are a healthcare hero.

Yes, you.

Now you have some skills and ideas for making the world a better place for anyone with an "oh damn" diagnosis. That means you're making healthcare less lonely and more inclusive for all feelings, not just the go-fight-win kind.

You're a platitude-killer and a support-warrior. You're a sounding board and logistics pro. You're a good friend and a good person.

Now, go be a teacher. Show everyone in your patient circle and beyond how to truly support someone who's sick. And if you should ever be sick, too, know that you're not alone. Not with all these healthcare heroes supporting us.